AVOID EATING PORK

WHITLEY SMITH

Copyright ©2020

TABLE OF CONTENT

INTRODUCTION

Particularly common in Europe, Oceania, Sub-Saharan Africa, North, and South America, and Eastern and Southern Asia, Pork is a generally consumed meat.

Pigs were regarded as the refuse, usually consuming virtually whatever they could obtain which comprises bugs, insects, remnants, their own defecation, and carcasses. Pigs are dirty animals, regardless of how you choose to view them.

It's important to know about pork as a meat prior to settling one's mind to consuming it.

Simply understanding **what a pig's diet entails**

might likewise clarify why the meat of the animal

could not be pleasant to eat.

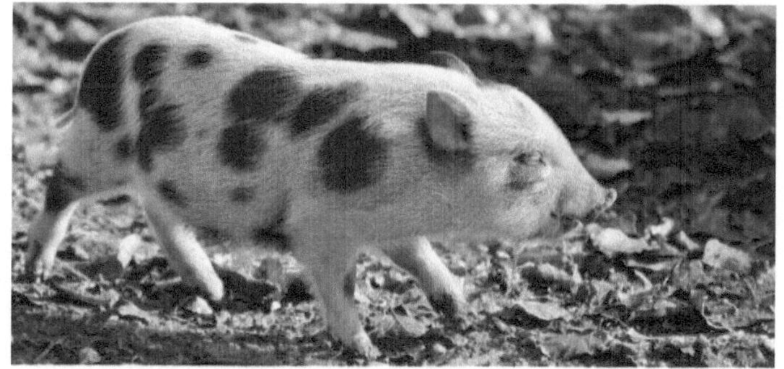

THE PIG DIGESTIVE SYSTEM

The sweat gland is renowned for assisting the body in sweating off impurities. It is important **to note that pigs have few sweat glands,** which makes it challenging for them to perspire. More toxins are left in the pig's body as a result. Therefore, all of these toxins that weren't removed are present in the pork meat when it is consumed.

The pig's fast-acting digestive tract prevents it from getting rid of the excess toxin and other potentially harmful meal ingredients. Because a pig can digest its food intake in four hours whereas it may take some other animals up to twelve or twenty-four hours to do so, those harmful toxins

remain in the pig's system and are later consumed

by humans who eat the meat.

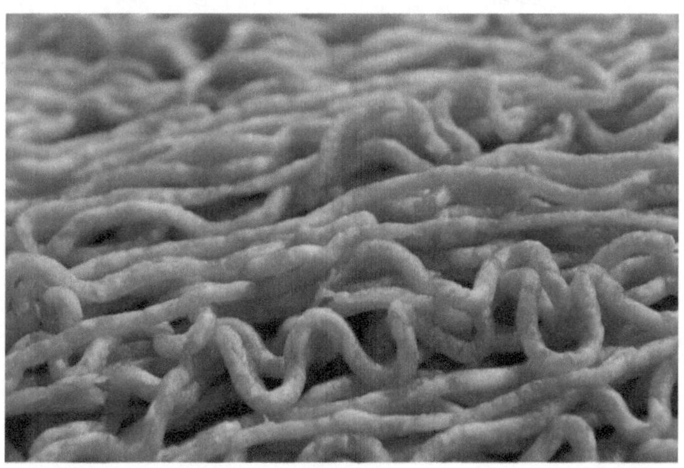

PIGS AND COMMON VIRUSES AND PARASITES

A lot of viruses and parasites are carried by pigs. Humans increase their likelihood of getting one of these terrible, frequently crippling diseases by coming into physical touch with them through farmland or by consuming their meat.

Pigs are primary carriers of:

- Nipah virus

- Taenia solium tapeworm

- Hepatitis E virus (HEV)

- Viruses in the family Paramyxoviridae

> ➢ Porcine reproductive and respiratory

> ➢ syndrome

> ➢ Menangle virus

Every one of these viruses and parasites has the possibility of causing severe medical conditions that may persist for decades.

Hepatitis E and Pork

Pork **liver is the primary food-based carrier of the Hepatitis E virus**, which affect millions of people every year and can cause illness, in advanced countries.

A proven hepatitis E carrier is France's native figatellu, a pork liver dish that is usually taken uncooked. Around 50% of the native community in areas in France where uncooked or barbecued pork is a typical cuisine exhibits signs of hepatitis E disease.

Roughly One out of every ten shop-bought pig livers in America test positive for hepatitis E, a figure that is greater than the one out of fifteen rates in the Netherlands and the one in twenty rates in the Czech Republic. In Germany, research revealed that about one out of five pig slaughters were infected.

Most hepatitis E infections are often symptom-free, however, pregnant women can suffer serious effects of the virus, involving fast organ damage and an elevated likelihood of mother and child death.

Mothers who contract the disease in their third trimester actually have a death rate that can be up to 25%. Hepatitis E infection might, in exceptional situations, cause inflammatory cardiovascular disease, acute pancreatitis, brain abnormalities, blood disorders, and nerve conditions.

Those with weaker immune systems, including those living with HIV, are more susceptible to suffering from this serious hepatitis E symptoms.

It could be natural to attribute the hepatitis E outbreak to industrial farming practices, however in the context of the pig, untamed does not correspond to healthier. Hepatitis E, which can create serious problems and even death in susceptible individuals, is usually present in pork products, especially in liver. Cooking is required to eliminate the virus.

Multiple Sclerosis and Pork

Multiple sclerosis, a debilitating auto-immune illness affecting the central nervous system, is one of the most unexpected risks linked to pork and one that has attracted little to no publicity. At least since researchers examined the relationship between per capita pork intake and Multiple Sclerosis across numerous nations, the connection between pork and Multiple Sclerosis has been recognized.

Although countries that are against Pork consumption, such as Israel, were mostly exempt from Multiple sclerosis's discriminatory grasps, open-minded consumers, like the United States of America suffered high rates.

Although a causal role for pork in multiple sclerosis is far from established, further research is necessary due to unexpectedly powerful epidemiological trends, scientific validity, and recorded occurrences.

Liver Cancer and Cirrhosis

Hepatitis B and C disease, aflatoxin, and too much alcohol are among the factors that are known to increase the risk for liver problems. Yet, there is another prospective threat to liver health that is concealed in scientific papers. Pork intake has continuously increased liver cancer and cirrhosis rates worldwide for years.

But pork-transmitted hepatitis E can cause liver cirrhosis; this occurs almost solely in individuals with a weak immune system.

In comparison to other meat, pork is often greater in omega-6 fatty acids, such as linoleic and arachidonic, which could have an impact on liver disease.

Heterocyclic amino acids, a group of carcinogens produced by cooking meat at extreme temps, aid in the creation of liver cancer in a wide range of animals. Yet, these substances are also mainly constituted in beef, according to to comparable research showing that pork has no strong association with liver illness. Given all of that in the account, it would be simple to write off the pig liver disease relationship as an epidemiological anomaly.

But there are a few logical processes that do happen. The most likely competitor includes nitrosamines, which are carcinogenic mixtures produced when nitrites and nitrates interact with specific amino acids especially when there is high heat. These component has been associated with damage and cancer in a number of different organs, as well as the liver.

Large amounts of nitrosamines have been discovered in ham, sausage, bacon, and other preserved meats. Bacon is a uniquely excellent source since the fatty portion of pork products appears to collect significantly greater levels of nitrosamines than the lean bits. Combining pork with vegetables may not provides much safety because the existence of fat could also turn vitamin C into a nitrosamine promoter rather than a blocker.

Despite the fact that most of the studies investigating the connection between nitrosamines and liver cancer have concentrated on rats, in which some nitrosamines can swiftly damage the liver, the impact also manifests in people. However, some experts contend that humans could be more susceptible to nitrosamines than rodents.

While there is currently insufficient data to conclusively link smoking, liver-damaging substances, and liver disease, the risk is reasonable enough to suggest restricting nitrosamine pork products, such as bacon, ham, and hot dogs made with potassium nitrate or sodium nitrite.

Pork Derived Food Product and Cancer

People who do the keto diet and other weight loss diets, however, mainly eat pig and processed meat.

They had no idea that eating foods like ham, sausage, and bacon was doing more damage to their health than good.

The World Health Organization claims that processed meat increases the risk of cancer. Processed meat is listed as a carcinogen by the International Agency for Research on Cancer.

Foods like ham, bacon, and sausage, which are mostly made from pig, are examples of processed meat.

Trichinosis and Pork

Trichinosis is among the main worries associated with eating pork. **Humans can contract this infection by consuming pork that has been half-done or not cooked at all and has been infested**

with trichinella worm larvae. Pork is a very popular host to this parasite. The worm's larvae are introduced into the pig's system when it breaks due to stomach acids.

These young worms settle in the muscles of the pig. Then, the unaware human body eats this diseased pork flesh. These worms have the same potential to harm humans as they do to pigs. If you consume fresh or half-done pork that is infected with the parasite, you will also be ingesting cyst-encased trichinella larvae. After some time, the larvae can travel to the bloodstream.

Trichinosis is a terrible disease that you ought to dodohatever to prevent.

Unusual signs may begin between one and two days following an infection, whereas other symptoms often appear between two and eight weeks following the infection.

According to the study, the degree to which the symptoms are severe primarily relies on how many larvae were absorbed in the contaminated meat. To get rid of any worms, it is advised to refrigerate the pork before cooking thoroughly.

Symptoms of Trichinosis

- ✓ Headache

- ✓ High fever

- ✓ Muscle pain and tenderness

- ✓ Pink eye

- ✓ Sensitivity to light

- ✓ Swelling of the eyelids or face

- ✓ General weakness

FACTORY FARMING AND PIGS

It is crucial that people are aware that one of the common conditions of pork bred for consumption is that pigs are occasionally raised with the intention of making money.

Factory farming is a **practice of rearing rapidly expanding animals in conditions of intense isolation, often to the level where the animals are unable to walk around.**

In factory farming, animals are **handled like instruments**. They are abused in various ways since the company sees them just as a means of making a gain. Gestation crates are frequently used to house pregnant pigs.

A surprising number of pigs in the United States are raised in factories nowadays.

In other words, these pigs never have a healthy life that includes clean air and wide-open spaces.

If you consume pork, you ought to be aware that you are probably consuming the flesh of a pig who had his whole life in confined spaces with little opportunity for clean air and has been fed a diet consisting of dangerous chemicals to keep it alive. These substances frequently cause the pigs to be curled under the weight increase that they have

acquired inappropriately and aggressively.

As a result, factory farming harms humans as well

as animals. People's health is another area where it

suffers. This is why you should stay away from

meat that has been raised in factories, especially

pork.

Awful Treatment of Pigs

Pigs are kept in gestation crates during pregnancy,

which, at just two feet wide, are not large enough

for them to move around or indulge in any natural

behaviors. The effects of this abhorrent abuse on a

pig's mental condition are summed up as follows by the Humane Society of the United States:

They bite on the bars, swing their heads unevenly back and forth, or rest unmoving on the ground. The pigs spend months expecting to be served after becoming virtually incapacitated, possibly breaking down in the process.

Afterward, their offspring are removed, the pigs are made pregnant again, and they are transferred to gestation crates to begin the full cycle of distress reproduction. Fortunately, many main food corporations are now promising to cease purchasing animals produced in this abhorrent manner as a result of the aggressive action taken by organizations like the Humane Society. The shift away from this disgusting policy will require time to fully execute, though.

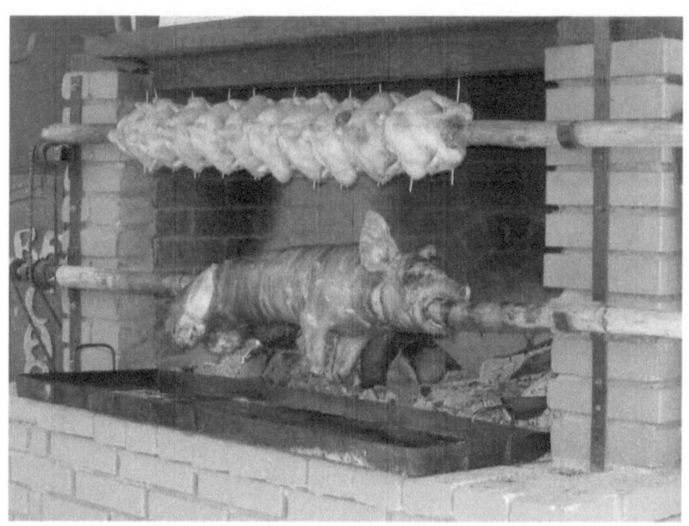

CONCLUSION

For its excessive use of antibiotics, a behavior that is adding to a national public health problem, the production of pork is infamous. The consequence could be that the antibiotics you or a loved one might require to fight an illness someday may not be effective. Pig farming is by far the biggest threat, using four times as much antibiotics per pound of meat as raising livestock and substantially more than chicken production, according to research conducted.

The pig's fast-acting digestive tract prevents it from getting rid of the excess toxin and other potentially harmful meal ingredients. Because a pig can digest its food intake in four hours whereas it may take some other animals up to twelve or twenty-four hours to do so, those harmful toxins remain in the pig's system and are later consumed by humans who eat the meat.

It's important to know about pork as a meat prior to settling one's mind to consuming it.

Simply understanding what a pig's diet entails might likewise clarify why the meat of the animal could not be pleasant to eat.

This is why you should stay away from meat that has been raised in factories, especially pork.